Table of Contents

Chapter 1: Introduction to Wound Care Nursing

- Definition and scope of wound care nursing
- Importance of wound care in healthcare
- Overview of common types of wounds

Chapter 2: Anatomy and Physiology of Skin

- Structure and function of the skin
- Stages of wound healing
- Factors affecting wound healing

Chapter 3: Assessing Wounds

- Initial wound assessment techniques
- Tools and technologies in wound assessment
- Documenting and charting wound progress

Chapter 4: Types of Wounds

- Acute vs. chronic wounds
- Common types of wounds (pressure ulcers, diabetic foot ulcers, venous ulcers, surgical wounds, traumatic wounds)
- Case studies

Chapter 5: Principles of Wound Management

- Cleansing and debridement
- Creating a moist wound environment
- Managing infection and inflammation

Chapter 6: Dressings and Wound Care Products

- Overview of dressing types and their applications
- Advances in wound care materials (hydrocolloids, foam dressings, alginates, etc.)
- Product selection based on wound type and stage

Chapter 7: Advanced Wound Care Techniques

- Negative pressure wound therapy (NPWT)
- Hyperbaric oxygen therapy
- Bioengineered skin and tissue products

Chapter 8: Pain Management in Wound Care

- Understanding pain in wound care patients
- Pharmacological and non-pharmacological pain management strategies
- Patient education on pain management

Chapter 9: Nutritional Considerations in Wound Healing

- Nutrition's role in wound healing
- Nutritional assessments and interventions

- Case studies on nutrition management

Chapter 10: Ethical and Legal Considerations in Wound Care

- Ethical dilemmas in wound care nursing
- Legal aspects of wound care treatment and documentation
- Case law and precedent in wound care

Chapter 11: Interprofessional Wound Care Team

- Roles and responsibilities of the wound care team
- Importance of interprofessional collaboration
- Case studies of successful team management

Chapter 12: Patient Education and Home Care

- Educating patients and caregivers
- Developing effective home care plans
- Utilizing community resources for wound care

Appendices

- Quick reference charts for wound types and care options
- Glossary of terms

About the Author

- Professional background
- Other publications
- Contact information

Disclaimer for "Advanced Wound Care: Techniques and Management" by Chad Peterson

The information provided in "Advanced Wound Care: Techniques and Management" is intended for educational purposes only and is not meant to replace professional medical advice, diagnosis, or treatment. While the content within this book is provided with the intent to offer accurate and up-to-date information regarding the topics discussed, the rapidly evolving nature of medical science means that new research and data may emerge following publication.

Readers are encouraged to consult a qualified healthcare provider for diagnosis and answers to their personal medical questions. No part of this publication should be interpreted as a tool for self-diagnosis or self-treatment. The application of any of the strategies, techniques, and recommendations presented in this book should be made based on professional judgment in consideration of individual patient conditions and circumstances.

Neither the author nor the publisher assumes any liability for any injury and/or damage to persons or property arising from this publication. The use of this book does not guarantee any specific patient outcome or response, and it should be used in conjunction with other professional resources and judgment.

By using this book, the reader agrees to the terms of this disclaimer and acknowledges that the authors and publishers are not responsible for any errors, omissions, or outcomes related to the use of the information provided herein.

Chapter 1: Introduction to Wound Care Nursing

Learning Objectives

By the end of this chapter, you will be able to:

1. Define wound care nursing and understand its critical role within healthcare.

2. Recognize the importance of wound care in improving patient outcomes.

3. Identify common types of wounds encountered in clinical practice.

4. Apply a holistic, client-centered, and evidence-based care model to wound care.

Definition and Scope of Wound Care Nursing

Wound care nursing is a specialized area of healthcare focused on the management and treatment of wounds that are chronic or hard to heal. This includes surgical wounds, ulcers, burns, and traumatic injuries. Wound care nurses play a pivotal role in preventing infection, promoting healing, and helping maintain patient comfort and mobility.

Importance of Wound Care in Healthcare

Effective wound care is essential not only for the healing of the wound itself but also for preventing potential complications such as infections and amputations. The expertise of wound care nurses is vital in managing the complexities of wound healing, which involves understanding the healing process, choosing appropriate treatment modalities, and considering the patient's overall health status.

Overview of Common Types of Wounds

- **Pressure Ulcers:** Often occur in patients who are immobile or bedridden, where constant pressure on certain areas leads to skin breakdown.

- **Diabetic Ulcers:** Commonly found on the feet of people with diabetes, these ulcers form due to impaired sensation and blood flow.

- **Venous Ulcers:** Typically located on the legs and caused by venous insufficiency, these ulcers are due to poor blood flow back to the heart.

- **Arterial Ulcers:** Result from inadequate blood flow to the limb, causing the skin and tissues to receive insufficient oxygen.

- **Surgical Wounds:** These can become problematic due to infection or poor surgical technique and require careful monitoring.

- **Traumatic Wounds:** Caused by an external force, these wounds vary in severity and type, such as abrasions, lacerations, or punctures.

Applying a Holistic, Client-Centered, and Evidence-Based Care Model

In wound care, a holistic approach takes into account all aspects of the patient's health and well-being. Treatment plans are client-centered, developed through partnerships between patients and healthcare providers and tailored to each patient's unique needs and circumstances. Evidence-based practice is critical, involving the integration of the best available research with clinical expertise and patient values.

Summary of Lessons Learned

- Wound care nursing is essential for effective healthcare delivery, requiring specialized knowledge and skills.

- Understanding different types of wounds allows for better planning and application of treatment strategies.

- Implementing a holistic, client-centered, and evidence-based approach enhances patient care and outcomes.

References

- Smith, J. (Year). ***Comprehensive Guide to Wound Care***. Medical Press.

- Doe, A., & Roe, B. (Year). ***Evidence-Based Wound Management***. Healing Publications.

This chapter sets the foundation for understanding the critical role of wound care nursing within the healthcare system, highlighting the importance of specialized care for different wound types and the benefits of employing a holistic and evidence-based approach to patient care.

Chapter 2: Anatomy and Physiology of Skin

Learning Objectives

By the end of this chapter, you will be able to:

1. Describe the structure and function of the skin in relation to overall health and wound healing.

2. Identify and explain the stages of wound healing.

3. Analyze various factors that can affect the process of wound healing.

4. Apply a holistic, client-centered, and evidence-based approach to managing and supporting wound healing.

Structure and Function of the Skin

The skin, the largest organ of the human body, serves as a protective barrier against mechanical impacts, pathogens, and environmental factors. It also plays crucial roles in sensation, temperature regulation, and the production of vitamin D. Structurally, the skin is divided into three primary layers:

- **Epidermis:** The outermost layer, providing barrier function and skin tone.

- **Dermis:** Beneath the epidermis, containing tough connective tissue, hair follicles, and sweat glands.

- **Hypodermis (subcutaneous layer):** Consists of fat and connective tissue that houses larger blood vessels and nerves, crucial for insulating and protecting the body's inner organs.

Stages of Wound Healing

Wound healing is a complex process that can be divided into four distinct stages:

1. **Hemostasis Phase:** Immediately after an injury, this phase involves blood clotting.
2. **Inflammatory Phase:** This phase cleans out the wound, involving swelling and redness as the body works to fight infection.
3. **Proliferative Phase:** The focus is on covering the wound with new tissue (granulation tissue) and developing new blood vessels.
4. **Maturation Phase:** The final stage where collagen is remodeled and the new tissue gains strength and flexibility.

Hemostasis Phase

- This initial phase begins immediately after an injury occurs and is crucial for stopping the bleeding. The body's response is to form a clot which not only reduces blood loss but also provides the initial matrix for subsequent healing stages. Blood vessels constrict to minimize blood flow, platelets stick together to form a clot, and a fibrin mesh is created to stabilize the clot which acts as a temporary barrier for the wound.

2. **Inflammatory Phase**

    o   Following hemostasis, the inflammatory phase kicks in, typically lasting a few days. This phase is characterized by redness, warmth, swelling, and pain at the wound site. These symptoms occur as the body's immune system sends white blood cells and nutrients to the area to fight infection and begin the healing process. During this phase, macrophages (a type of white blood cell) not only help clean the wound by phagocytizing debris and pathogens but also release growth factors that are critical for the healing process.

3. **Proliferative Phase**

    o   The third phase is the proliferative phase, where the focus shifts to covering and strengthening the wound. This phase can last several weeks and involves three major processes: fibroplasia or the formation of granulation tissue, angiogenesis or the formation of new blood vessels, and epithelialization, where new skin cells spread across the surface of the wound to cover it. Granulation tissue, which is rich in collagen and has a distinct red, bumpy look, forms the foundation of new tissue. Meanwhile, new blood vessels are essential to supply nutrients and oxygen that are critical for continued healing.

4. **Maturation Phase**

    o   Also known as the remodeling phase, this is the final stage of wound healing. It can start around three weeks after the injury and last for months or even years. In this phase, the collagen that was hastily laid down in the proliferative phase is now remodeled to increase the tensile strength of the wound. The new tissue, initially a scar, gradually becomes stronger and more flexible. The number of blood vessels in the area decreases, which causes the red color of the granulation tissue to fade.

Understanding these stages helps healthcare providers manage wounds effectively, ensuring that interventions support the natural healing process at each stage. This knowledge is crucial for developing treatment plans that address the specific needs of the wound at each phase of healing.

NURSING CONSIDERATIONS

For each stage of the wound healing process, nursing considerations play a crucial role in ensuring effective care and optimal outcomes. Nurses must be attentive to the needs of the wound and the patient, adjusting their interventions based on the healing stage and individual patient factors. Here are some key nursing considerations for each stage of wound healing:

1. **Hemostasis Phase**

    - **Immediate Care:** Nurses should promptly assess the wound for severity, control bleeding, and prevent further injury or contamination. This involves applying pressure, using appropriate wound dressings, and maintaining sterile techniques.

    - **Assessment:** Continuous monitoring for signs of excessive bleeding or hematoma formation is crucial. Ensuring that the patient maintains adequate hemodynamic stability is also important.

    - **Education:** Educate the patient and family on the importance of keeping the wound clean and protected, and advise on recognizing signs of complications such as increased bleeding.

2. **Inflammatory Phase**

- **Infection Prevention:** Regular cleaning of the wound, changing dressings as needed, and observing for signs of infection (e.g., increased redness, pus, odor, or unusual swelling) are critical. Use of prophylactic antibiotics should be considered as per the healthcare provider's prescription.

- **Pain Management:** Manage pain through appropriate analgesics and non-pharmacological methods like elevation of the injured area to reduce swelling.

- **Nutritional Support:** Encourage a diet high in proteins, vitamins (particularly A and C), and minerals like zinc to support the immune system and aid in healing.

3. **Proliferative Phase**

    - **Wound Care:** Continue with regular cleaning and dressing changes. Use moisture-retentive dressings to promote granulation and epithelialization. Avoid disrupting the wound bed to protect new granulation tissue.

    - **Monitoring for Adequate Healing:** Assess for signs of healthy new tissue formation and ensure that the wound is contracting properly. Monitor for any signs of hypertrophic scarring.

    - **Patient Education:** Teach the patient about the signs of healthy healing versus signs of complications, and instruct on continued care of the wound at home.

4. **Maturation Phase**

    - **Long-term Care:** Continue to protect the new scar tissue from injury and monitor for any changes in the scar appearance. Advise on the use of sunscreen to protect the new skin from UV damage.

- **Scar Management:** Depending on the location and severity of the scar, consider interventions such as silicone gel sheets, massage, or other therapies to improve the appearance and flexibility of the scar.

- **Rehabilitation:** If the wound is extensive, involve physical therapy to prevent contractures and ensure proper mobility.

Throughout all stages, maintaining a holistic approach is vital. This includes considering the patient's overall health status, comorbidities (like diabetes or vascular diseases that could impair healing), and psychological wellbeing. Effective communication, meticulous documentation, and collaboration with the rest of the healthcare team are essential to ensure comprehensive wound management and care.

Factors Affecting Wound Healing

Several factors can influence how effectively a wound heals:

- **Nutritional Status:** Adequate nutrition, particularly protein and vitamin C, is crucial for effective healing.

- **Blood Flow and Oxygenation:** Good circulation is essential to supply oxygen and nutrients to the wound.

- **Infection:** Infections can delay healing by damaging new tissue and causing inflammation.

- **Age:** Older age can slow down the healing process due to reduced skin elasticity and slower cellular activity.

- **Smoking:** Smoking impairs blood flow and oxygenation, significantly affecting wound healing.

- **Chronic Diseases:** Conditions like diabetes or vascular disease can impair healing due to poor blood flow and other complications.

The factors that affect wound healing are critical in determining the treatment and care approach for effective recovery. Understanding these factors can help nurses tailor their interventions and patient education to optimize wound healing. Below, I will expand on these factors, including specific nursing considerations and client education strategies:

1. **Nutritional Status**

   - **Nursing Considerations:** Assess the patient's dietary intake and nutritional status regularly. If necessary, collaborate with a dietitian to provide a high-protein, high-vitamin diet tailored to the patient's needs. Monitor albumin and prealbumin levels as indicators of nutritional status.

   - **Client Education:** Educate patients on the importance of a balanced diet rich in protein, vitamins A and C, and zinc to support wound healing. Encourage hydration and discuss the impact of nutrition on recovery.

2. **Blood Flow and Oxygenation**

   - **Nursing Considerations:** Assess circulation in areas around the wound. Use interventions such as positioning, gentle exercise (as appropriate), and avoiding restrictive clothing or devices to improve blood flow. Monitor for signs of decreased perfusion or oxygenation.

- **Client Education:** Teach patients about the importance of regular movement to enhance circulation, avoiding long periods of inactivity, and the significance of not smoking to maintain good blood flow.

3. **Infection**

    - **Nursing Considerations:** Keep the wound clean and dry. Use sterile techniques for dressing changes. Monitor the wound closely for signs of infection such as increased redness, swelling, heat, pain, or discharge, and initiate appropriate antimicrobial treatments as prescribed.

    - **Client Education:** Instruct patients on how to care for their wound at home, recognize signs of infection, and understand when to seek medical help. Emphasize the importance of hand hygiene before and after touching the wound.

4. **Age**

    - **Nursing Considerations:** Pay extra attention to the skin integrity of older adults. Provide gentle care and consider the use of skin protectants and appropriate moisturizers to maintain skin health.

    - **Client Education:** Discuss with older patients and their caregivers the expectations for slower healing times and the importance of regular check-ups to monitor wound progress.

5. **Smoking**

- **Nursing Considerations:** Encourage patients who smoke to participate in smoking cessation programs. Monitor for any complications associated with reduced oxygenation.

- **Client Education:** Educate patients on how smoking adversely affects wound healing by constricting blood vessels and reducing oxygen supply to the tissues, and discuss available resources for quitting smoking.

6. **Chronic Diseases**

    - **Nursing Considerations:** For patients with chronic conditions like diabetes or vascular diseases, closely monitor blood glucose levels, manage underlying conditions, and coordinate care with other healthcare providers.

    - **Client Education:** Teach patients with chronic diseases about how their condition affects wound healing. Stress the importance of managing their chronic condition to improve healing outcomes, such as controlling blood sugar in diabetics or improving vascular health in those with circulatory issues.

Applying a Holistic, Client-Centered, and Evidence-Based Care Model

Effective wound management requires a comprehensive approach that considers all aspects of a patient's health and lifestyle. By understanding and addressing the individual needs and conditions that might affect wound healing, healthcare providers can develop personalized, effective care plans. Employing evidence-based practices ensures that these plans are grounded in the latest research and best practices, optimizing outcomes.

Summary of Lessons Learned

- The skin's complex structure plays an integral role in protecting the body and supporting wound healing.
- The healing process is dynamic and can be influenced by a wide range of internal and external factors.
- A holistic, patient-centered approach to care is crucial in effectively managing wound healing.

References

- Brown, M. & Edwards, H. (Year). *Skin Integrity and Wound Care Management*. Elsevier Health Sciences.
- Lee, C.Y. & Kozol, R. (Year). *Factors Affecting Wound Healing*. Journal of Wound Care.

This chapter provides a foundational understanding of the anatomy and physiology of the skin and outlines the stages and factors affecting wound healing, emphasizing the importance of a holistic, evidence-based approach to optimizing patient recovery and health outcomes.

Chapter 3: Assessing Wounds

Learning Objectives

By the end of this chapter, you will be able to:

1. Execute initial wound assessments using standardized techniques.

2. Utilize various tools and technologies effectively in wound assessment.

3. Implement thorough and consistent documentation practices to chart wound progress.

4. Apply a holistic, client-centered, and evidence-based approach to wound assessment.

Initial Wound Assessment Techniques

Wound assessment is a critical first step in effective wound management. An initial assessment should include a detailed examination of the wound's location, size, depth, and the condition of the surrounding skin. It is also important to assess for signs of infection and any potential complications. Key elements of initial wound assessment include:

- **Visual Inspection:** Observing the wound for color, size, and signs of healing or complications.

- **Palpation:** Feeling around the wound for temperature, consistency, and to assess pain.

- **Exudate Assessment:** Evaluating the amount and type of exudate (fluid) the wound is producing, which can indicate the stage of healing or infection.

Proper assessment of a wound is crucial for determining its stage of healing, identifying complications, and guiding effective management strategies. The primary methods for assessing a wound include visual inspection, palpation, and exudate assessment. Below, I'll expand on these techniques along with specific nursing considerations:

1. **Visual Inspection**

    - **Process:** Visual inspection involves carefully examining the wound for changes in size, color, and general appearance. This includes noting the presence of granulation tissue (red, bumpy appearance indicating healing), necrotic tissue (black or brown tissue that needs to be removed), and any signs of infection such as increased redness or purulent discharge.

    - **Nursing Considerations:** Nurses should ensure adequate lighting and use a ruler or measuring tape to track changes in wound size. Photographs may be taken (with patient consent) to document progress. It's essential to compare the current state of the wound with previous assessments to monitor healing or worsening.

    - **Documentation:** Document all findings accurately in the patient's medical record, including descriptions of the wound's size, depth, color, and any other notable characteristics. This documentation is vital for tracking healing over time and communicating with other healthcare providers.

2. **Palpation**

- **Process:** Palpation involves gently pressing around and, if appropriate, directly on the wound to assess characteristics such as temperature (warmth may indicate infection), consistency (softness, firmness, induration), and pain. It helps in evaluating the extent of the injury, including possible involvement of underlying structures.

- **Nursing Considerations:** Nurses should use gloves to maintain sterility and possibly anesthetic sprays or creams if the palpation causes pain. It's important to be gentle to avoid causing additional trauma to the wound or discomfort to the patient.

- **Documentation:** Record findings like tenderness, warmth, or induration, as these can indicate infection or other complications. Also, note the patient's response to palpation, as significant pain might necessitate further evaluation or adjustment of pain management strategies.

3. **Exudate Assessment**

    - **Process:** Assessing the amount and type of exudate (fluid produced by the wound) is critical. Different types of exudate, such as serous (clear, watery), purulent (thick, yellow, green, or brown, indicating infection), or sanguineous (containing blood), provide information about the wound's condition and the healing stage.

    - **Nursing Considerations:** Use appropriate absorbent materials to collect and measure exudate if necessary. Adjust wound dressings based on the amount of exudate: more absorbent dressings for heavy exudate and moisture-retaining dressings for wounds with less or no exudate to promote a moist healing environment.

- **Documentation:** Document the type, color, odor, and quantity of exudate. Changes in exudate characteristics can be significant indicators of healing progression or emerging complications, such as infection or dehiscence (wound reopening).

Overall Nursing Approach: Incorporating these assessment techniques requires a systematic approach and attention to detail. Nurses must be vigilant and responsive to any changes observed through these methods. Effective communication with the healthcare team and ongoing education of the patient and family about the significance of these findings are also critical components of comprehensive wound care. By maintaining a thorough assessment regimen, nurses play a pivotal role in facilitating optimal wound healing and preventing complications.

Tools and Technologies in Wound Assessment

Advancements in technology have enhanced the precision and efficiency of wound assessments. Some commonly used tools include:

- **Digital Photography:** Allows for consistent visual monitoring and aids in documenting healing progress.

- **Wound Measurement Tools:** Devices like calipers or rulers used to provide accurate measurements of wound dimensions.

- **Tissue Oxygenation Monitors:** Non-invasive devices that measure the level of oxygen available to the wound, important for healing.

- **Thermal Imaging Cameras:** Detect changes in skin temperature around the wound, which can indicate infection or inflammation.

Documenting and Charting Wound Progress

Effective documentation is crucial in wound care for tracking the healing process, facilitating communication among care providers, and ensuring continuity of care. Essential aspects of documenting wound progress include:

- **Wound Charts:** Detailed charts including size, depth, and characteristics of the wound over time.

- **Photographic Records:** Regularly updated photos to visually track healing.

- **Notes on Patient Feedback:** Including patient's reports of pain and other symptoms, which can provide insights into the healing process or emerging complications.

Wound Charting Template

Patient Information:

- Name: _____
- Date of Birth: _____
- Medical Record Number: _____
- Date of Admission: _____

- **Location of Wound(s):** _____

Wound Assessment:

1. **Date of Assessment:**
   - Date: _____

2. **Type of Wound:**
   - Pressure Ulcer
   - Diabetic Foot Ulcer
   - Venous Ulcer
   - Surgical Wound
   - Traumatic Wound
   - Burn

3. **Wound Location:**
   - _____

4. **Wound Size:**
   - Length: _____ cm
   - Width: _____ cm
   - Depth: _____ cm

5. **Wound Appearance:**
   - Necrotic Tissue

- Slough
- Granulation Tissue
- Epithelializing
- Closed

6. **Wound Edges:**

   - Attached
   - Unattached
   - Undermining (specify extent): _____
   - Maceration

7. **Exudate:**

   - None
   - Scant
   - Moderate
   - Copious
   - Type (serous, purulent, etc.): _____

8. **Odor:**

   - None
   - Present (describe): _____

9. **Pain Assessment:**

   - None

- o Mild
- o Moderate
- o Severe
- o Description of pain (continuous, intermittent): _____

10. Surrounding Skin:

- o Intact
- o Erythema
- o Induration
- o Warmth
- o Other abnormalities: _____

Treatment Provided:

- **Topical Treatments:**
  - o Type of dressing applied: _____
  - o Medications applied: _____
  - o Cleansing solutions used: _____

- **Systemic Treatments:**
  - o Antibiotics
  - o Analgesics
  - o Other medications: _____

- **Other Interventions:**
    - Debridement
    - Negative Pressure Wound Therapy
    - Surgery
    - Other: _____

Patient and Caregiver Education:

- Provided on date: _____
- Topics covered: _____
- Educational materials given: _____
- Follow-up education needed: _____

Plan and Goals:

- **Short-term goals:**
    - _____

- **Long-term goals:**
    - _____

Next Assessment Date:

- _____

Nurse/Healthcare Provider Signature:

- _____

Applying a Holistic, Client-Centered, and Evidence-Based Care Model

In wound assessment, integrating a holistic and client-centered approach involves considering the entire well-being of the patient, including physical, emotional, and social factors that might impact wound healing. Using evidence-based guidelines ensures that assessments are accurate and treatments are appropriately tailored to each patient's unique needs.

Summary of Lessons Learned

- Accurate and thorough initial assessments are vital for effective wound management.

- Utilizing advanced tools and technologies can enhance the accuracy of wound assessments.

- Consistent and detailed documentation is crucial for monitoring healing progress and guiding treatment decisions.

References

- Jenkins, T. & Cooper, R. (Year). *Essentials of Wound Assessment*. Wound Care Alliance.

- Smith, G. (Year). *Modern Technologies in Wound Care*. TechMed Press.

This chapter outlines the importance of detailed and systematic wound assessment and the role of various tools and technologies in supporting these efforts. By embracing a holistic, client-centered, and evidence-based approach, healthcare providers can ensure comprehensive care and optimized outcomes for patients with wounds.

Chapter 4: Types of Wounds

Learning Objectives

By the end of this chapter, you will be able to:

1. Differentiate between acute and chronic wounds and understand their distinct characteristics.

2. Identify and describe the common types of wounds, including pressure ulcers, burns, diabetic foot ulcers, venous ulcers, surgical wounds, and traumatic wounds.

3. Analyze case studies to apply theoretical knowledge to practical scenarios.

4. Implement a holistic, client-centered, and evidence-based approach to managing various types of wounds.

Acute vs. Chronic Wounds

Understanding the difference between acute and chronic wounds is crucial for effective management:

- **Acute Wounds** occur as a result of surgery or trauma. They heal at a predictable and expected rate according to the normal wound healing process, which involves hemostasis, inflammation, proliferation, and maturation.

- **Chronic Wounds** fail to proceed through the normal stages of healing in a timely and orderly manner. These wounds often remain in the inflammatory phase and are usually associated with underlying conditions, such as diabetes or vascular disease.

Common Types of Wounds

Each type of wound requires specific management strategies:

- **Pressure Ulcers:** Also known as bedsores, these occur on skin that is under pressure for a prolonged period. Typically found on skin over bony areas.

- **Burns:** Caused by thermal, chemical, or electrical sources, burns are characterized by severe skin damage that causes the affected skin cells to die.

- **Diabetic Foot Ulcers:** Common in individuals with diabetes, these ulcers form as a result of skin tissue breaking down and exposing the layers underneath. They are often found under the big toes and on the balls of the feet.

- **Venous Ulcers:** These ulcers occur on the leg due to improper functioning of venous valves, often leading to increased venous pressure and edema which hinders proper skin nutrition.

- **Surgical Wounds:** Incisions or excisions that occur during surgery. They can become complicated by infection or poor healing.

- **Traumatic Wounds:** Result from any injury that causes skin disruption, including cuts, lacerations, or punctures.

Pressure Ulcers

Nursing Considerations:

- Regularly assess the skin, especially over bony prominences, for signs of pressure damage.

- Implement a turning schedule to relieve pressure.

Nursing Interventions:

- Use specialized mattresses or cushions to redistribute pressure.
- Keep the skin clean and dry to prevent infection.

Client Education:

- Educate clients and caregivers on the importance of regular repositioning and skin inspection.
- Discuss proper nutrition and hydration to support skin integrity.

Client Goal Setting:

- Set goals for regular position changes and skin assessments.
- Aim for gradual improvement or maintenance of skin condition without new ulcer formation.

2. Burns

Nursing Considerations:

- Assess burn severity and cover the area to prevent infection.
- Manage pain and prevent shock.

Nursing Interventions:

- Apply appropriate wound dressings and change them as needed.
- Provide fluid resuscitation as required.

Client Education:

- Teach clients about wound care, infection signs, and pain management.
- Advise on the importance of follow-up care for scar management.

Client Goal Setting:

- Establish pain management routines.
- Set benchmarks for wound healing and infection prevention.

3. Diabetic Foot Ulcers

Nursing Considerations:

- Regularly inspect feet for signs of injury or infection.
- Manage blood glucose levels to promote healing.

Nursing Interventions:

- Educate on proper foot care and hygiene.
- Use therapeutic footwear to reduce pressure on the ulcer.

Client Education:

- Stress the importance of daily foot inspections and wearing appropriate footwear.
- Discuss blood glucose management strategies.

Client Goal Setting:

- Set goals for consistent blood sugar control.
- Aim for timely healing of ulcers, with interventions adjusted based on progress.

4. Venous Ulcers

Nursing Considerations:

- Evaluate for signs of venous insufficiency like leg swelling and varicose veins.
- Use compression therapy to improve venous return.

Nursing Interventions:

- Apply compression stockings or bandages.
- Elevate legs to reduce edema.

Client Education:

- Explain the purpose and proper application of compression garments.
- Encourage mobility to enhance venous circulation.

Client Goal Setting:

- Establish a routine for leg elevation and compression garment use.
- Set realistic expectations for ulcer healing timeframes.

5. Surgical Wounds

Nursing Considerations:

- Monitor for signs of infection or dehiscence.
- Manage pain and support mobilization.

Nursing Interventions:

- Keep surgical sites clean and properly dressed.
- Encourage gentle activity as tolerated to promote circulation.

Client Education:

- Teach signs of infection and the importance of wound care.
- Discuss pain management options and the importance of activity.

Client Goal Setting:

- Aim for optimal pain control.
- Set milestones for wound closure and strength recovery.

6. Traumatic Wounds

Nursing Considerations:

- Cleanse wounds to remove debris and prevent infection.
- Assess for tetanus immunization status.

Nursing Interventions:

- Apply appropriate dressings and possibly administer tetanus prophylaxis.
- Manage pain and monitor for signs of infection.

Client Education:

- Instruct on wound care and signs of infection.
- Advise on updating tetanus vaccination if necessary.

Client Goal Setting:

- Goals for complete wound healing and infection prevention.
- Educate on methods to avoid future injuries.

General Considerations: In all cases, maintaining a clean environment, closely monitoring for signs of complications, and collaborating with a multidisciplinary team are crucial. Client education is integral for empowering patients to take an active role in their care, which significantly impacts outcomes. Setting clear, measurable goals with the client ensures that both patient and care provider are aligned and can track progress effectively.

Case Studies

Several case studies are presented to illustrate different wound types, their treatment strategies, and outcomes, providing practical insights into real-world clinical decision-making.

Case Study 1: Pressure Ulcer

Patient Profile:

- **Age/Gender:** 76/Male
- **Medical History:** Paralysis due to spinal cord injury, diabetes mellitus

Scenario: Mr. Smith, a wheelchair-bound patient, presented with a Stage III pressure ulcer on his sacrum, attributed to prolonged sitting and limited mobility.

Treatment Plan:

- **Initial Care:** Regular repositioning every 2 hours to alleviate pressure, use of a high-specification foam mattress.

- **Wound Care:** Application of a hydrocolloid dressing to maintain a moist healing environment and protect from infection.

- **Nutritional Support:** Enhanced protein intake and vitamin C supplementation to support skin repair and collagen formation.

- **Education:** Family was educated on the importance of repositioning and skin inspection routines.

Outcome: After 6 weeks, the ulcer showed signs of healing, with reduced size and increased granulation tissue. Continuous monitoring and care adjustments were planned to prevent recurrence.

Case Study 2: Diabetic Foot Ulcer

Patient Profile:

- **Age/Gender:** 58/Female

- **Medical History:** Type 2 diabetes, peripheral neuropathy

Scenario: Mrs. Gonzalez developed a non-healing foot ulcer on her heel, which she did not initially feel due to diabetic neuropathy.

Treatment Plan:

- **Wound Assessment:** Off-loading the foot using specialized diabetic footwear to reduce pressure.

- **Wound Management:** Daily saline cleansing and application of an alginate dressing to absorb excess exudate.

- **Diabetes Control:** Adjustment of her glycemic management regimen to optimize blood sugar levels.

- **Patient Education:** Instruction on daily foot care practices to prevent future injuries.

Outcome: The ulcer began to improve within a month, with proper glycemic control playing a crucial role. Mrs. Gonzalez continued with regular podiatry visits to prevent future complications.

Case Study 3: Venous Ulcer

Patient Profile:

- **Age/Gender:** 65/Male

- **Medical History:** Chronic venous insufficiency, obesity

Scenario: Mr. Johnson presented with a large, painful venous ulcer on his lower left leg, characterized by heavy exudate and surrounding skin erythema.

Treatment Plan:

- **Compression Therapy:** Application of multi-layer compression bandaging to improve venous return.

- **Wound Care:** Use of foam dressings to manage exudate and protect the surrounding skin.

- **Lifestyle Modifications:** Weight loss program to reduce leg pressure and improve overall vascular health.

- **Education:** Patient was educated on leg elevation techniques to use at home to decrease venous pressure.

Outcome: The ulcer size reduced significantly after 8 weeks of consistent compression therapy and improved lifestyle habits. Mr. Johnson was encouraged to continue with weight management and compression stockings.

Case Study 4: Burn Wound

Patient Profile:

- **Age/Gender:** 30/Male
- **Medical History:** No significant history

Scenario: Mr. Lee suffered second-degree burns on his forearm from a cooking oil accident at home.

Treatment Plan:

- **Immediate Care:** Cooling the burn under running water, assessing the severity.
- **Wound Care:** Application of silver sulfadiazine cream to prevent infection and facilitate healing.
- **Pain Management:** Over-the-counter pain relievers as needed.
- **Education:** Mr. Lee was educated on how to care for his burn and signs of infection to watch for during recovery.

Outcome: The burn healed without infection over several weeks, with Mr. Lee following up for potential scar management options.

These case studies provide practical examples of how different wound types require specialized approaches, reflecting the necessity of an individualized, holistic, and evidence-based care plan for optimal healing outcomes.

Applying a Holistic, Client-Centered, and Evidence-Based Care Model

Effective wound management involves not only understanding the type of wound but also considering the whole patient—lifestyle, co-morbidities, and social factors that could impact healing. Tailoring the wound care plan to each individual's circumstances ensures the best possible outcomes.

Summary of Lessons Learned

- Effective wound care management requires understanding the distinct characteristics of each wound type.
- A holistic approach that considers the entire well-being of the patient is essential for the effective healing of both acute and chronic wounds.
- Real-world case studies are valuable for understanding complex situations and enhancing decision-making skills.

References

- Black, J. & Hawk, J. (Year). *Clinical Management of Wounds*. Comprehensive Wound Care.
- White, S. & Mather, T. (Year). *Case Studies in Wound Care*. Wound Healing Society.

This chapter provides a comprehensive overview of different types of wounds, emphasizing the importance of categorizing them correctly and applying specific management principles. By integrating a holistic, client-centered, and evidence-based approach, healthcare providers can optimize wound care and improve patient outcomes.

Chapter 5: Principles of Wound Management

Learning Objectives

By the end of this chapter, you will be able to:

1. Execute effective wound cleansing and understand the importance of proper debridement.

2. Describe the methods to create and maintain a moist wound environment and explain its benefits in healing.

3. Identify strategies for managing infection and inflammation in wound care.

4. Integrate a holistic, client-centered, and evidence-based approach in managing wounds to optimize healing outcomes.

Cleansing and Debridement

Cleansing is crucial for removing contaminants and debris that could cause infection and delay healing. This section covers:

- **Techniques for Wound Cleansing:** Using appropriate solutions and methods to ensure effective cleaning without causing additional trauma to the wound bed.

- **Debridement Methods:** Describing surgical, autolytic, enzymatic, and mechanical debridement, focusing on how to choose the best method based on the wound's condition.

Techniques for Wound Cleansing

Purpose and Importance: Wound cleansing is vital to remove contaminants, exudate, and necrotic tissue, thereby reducing the risk of infection and promoting a healthy environment for healing.

Techniques:

- **Selection of Cleansing Solution:** Use non-toxic solutions like normal saline or prescribed antiseptic solutions. Avoid using cytotoxic agents like hydrogen peroxide or iodine solutions on chronic wounds, as they can damage granulation tissue.

- **Cleansing Method:** Gently irrigate the wound using a syringe to ensure adequate pressure to remove debris without causing trauma. For more fragile wounds, a soft gauze soaked in cleansing solution can be used to dab the wound gently.

Nursing Considerations:

- Assess the wound before and after cleansing to monitor changes and effectiveness of cleaning.

- Choose the cleansing technique based on the wound's condition and the amount of debris. Avoid aggressive scrubbing which can damage new tissue.

- Maintain sterile techniques to prevent introducing infections.

Patient Education:

- Educate patients on the importance of gentle, thorough wound cleaning to prevent infection and promote healing.

- Instruct on the signs of infection to watch for following cleansing.

Debridement Methods

Purpose and Importance: Debridement is crucial for removing non-viable tissue from the wound, which can harbor bacteria and delay healing.

Techniques:

1. **Surgical Debridement:**
   - The most immediate method for removing large amounts of necrotic tissue.
   - Performed by a trained professional using surgical instruments.

2. **Autolytic Debridement:**
   - Uses the body's own enzymes and moisture to liquefy dead tissue.
   - Achieved through moisture-retaining dressings like hydrogels or hydrocolloids.

3. **Enzymatic Debridement:**
   - Involves the application of topical enzymatic agents that break down necrotic tissue.
   - Specific to the type of tissue to be removed, and requires careful monitoring.

4. **Mechanical Debridement:**
   - Involves physical removal of dead tissue.
   - Techniques include wet-to-dry dressings, hydrotherapy, and wound irrigation.

Nursing Considerations:

- Carefully select debridement method based on the patient's overall health, wound characteristics, and pain tolerance.

- Monitor the wound and surrounding skin for any signs of irritation or adverse reactions during and after debridement.

- Manage pain effectively, as some methods, especially surgical and mechanical, can be painful.

Patient Education:

- Explain the purpose and process of each type of debridement to help the patient understand the importance of removing non-viable tissue.

- Discuss pain management options prior to procedures like surgical debridement.

Goal Setting with Patients:

- Set realistic goals for wound appearance and healing timelines after debridement.

- Engage patients in tracking progress towards these goals to maintain motivation and adherence to treatment plans.

By applying these wound cleansing and debridement techniques appropriately and considering each patient's individual needs, nurses can significantly influence the healing process, improve outcomes, and enhance patient satisfaction with their care.

Creating a Moist Wound Environment

Maintaining a moist environment is key to promoting faster and more effective healing. This part of the chapter explains:

- **Benefits of Moisture in Healing:** How maintaining moisture can enhance epithelialization and reduce pain.

- **Dressings and Products:** A review of various dressings such as hydrocolloids, hydrogels, foams, and alginates that help maintain optimal moisture levels.

Managing Infection and Inflammation

Infection and inflammation can severely impact wound healing. Effective management includes:

- **Recognizing Signs of Infection:** Learning to identify early signs of infection to prevent complications.

- **Anti-inflammatory Treatments:** Using pharmacological agents such as NSAIDs and corticosteroids, and non-pharmacological methods like proper nutrition and hydration.

- **Antimicrobial Stewardship:** Appropriate use of topical and systemic antibiotics to manage and prevent wound infections.

Managing infection and inflammation effectively is crucial for promoting optimal wound healing and preventing complications. Below is a detailed explanation of strategies for managing these issues, including nursing considerations, interventions, and patient education.

Recognizing Signs of Infection

Importance: Early recognition and intervention can prevent the progression of infection, which can impede healing processes and lead to more severe health issues.

Signs to Recognize:

- Increased redness around the wound
- Swelling or warmth
- Pus or malodorous discharge
- Pain or tenderness increases
- Fever or chills in the patient

Nursing Considerations:

- Conduct regular and thorough assessments of the wound during each dressing change.
- Use aseptic techniques to prevent introducing infections during wound care.

Nursing Interventions:

- Document and report any signs of infection immediately.
- Collect wound cultures if infection is suspected, before starting antibiotics.

Patient Education:

- Teach patients and caregivers how to identify signs of infection.
- Instruct on proper hand hygiene and wound care techniques to minimize infection risk.

Anti-inflammatory Treatments

Pharmacological Treatments:

- **NSAIDs:** Useful for reducing pain and inflammation. Must be used with caution, especially in patients with renal issues or gastrointestinal risks.

- **Corticosteroids:** May be used for severe inflammation but are generally avoided for long-term wound management due to potential side effects like delayed wound healing and increased infection risk.

Non-pharmacological Treatments:

- **Nutrition:** Ensure adequate intake of anti-inflammatory foods rich in omega-3 fatty acids, antioxidants, and proteins.

- **Hydration:** Maintain optimal hydration to support overall health and cellular functions essential for healing.

Nursing Considerations:

- Monitor patients for side effects of anti-inflammatory medications.

- Assess nutritional status and encourage dietary adjustments to support wound healing.

Nursing Interventions:

- Administer prescribed medications and monitor their effectiveness.

- Collaborate with dietitians to create a tailored nutrition plan.

Patient Education:

- Educate about the benefits and risks of NSAIDs and corticosteroids.

- Provide guidance on dietary choices that can naturally reduce inflammation.

Antimicrobial Stewardship

Purpose: To ensure the appropriate use of antimicrobials to treat infections without contributing to antibiotic resistance.

Approaches:

- **Topical Antibiotics:** Used directly on the wound to minimize systemic side effects.
- **Systemic Antibiotics:** Used when infection is severe or spreading beyond the wound.

Nursing Considerations:

- Evaluate the necessity and duration of antibiotic therapy to avoid overuse.
- Monitor for signs of allergic reactions or side effects from antibiotics.

Nursing Interventions:

- Administer antibiotics as prescribed and ensure adherence to the treatment regimen.
- Assess effectiveness and watch for any signs indicating the need for adjustment of therapy.

Patient Education:

- Explain the importance of completing the entire course of antibiotics even if symptoms improve.

- Discuss the risks of antibiotic resistance and the importance of using these medications only as directed.

Goal Setting with Patients:

- Set specific, measurable goals related to infection control, such as reduction in signs of infection and adherence to treatment plans.

- Regularly review these goals with patients and adjust care plans as needed to ensure progress.

Effective management of infection and inflammation through these strategies not only facilitates better wound healing but also enhances overall patient outcomes. Nurses play a pivotal role in implementing these strategies, monitoring their effectiveness, and educating patients to take an active role in managing their health.

Applying a Holistic, Client-Centered, and Evidence-Based Care Model

This section integrates holistic care by considering all aspects of the patient's health and lifestyle that affect wound healing. It emphasizes:

- **Personalized Care Plans:** Tailoring treatment strategies to individual needs, taking into account the patient's overall health, lifestyle, and preferences.

- **Collaborative Care:** Working with a multidisciplinary team to address the full spectrum of needs associated with wound management.

Summary of Lessons Learned

- Proper wound management involves meticulous cleansing, the right choice of debridement technique, maintaining a moist healing environment, and effective infection control.

- Applying a holistic and patient-centered approach enhances the effectiveness of treatment plans and supports better healing outcomes.

References

- Johnson, M. & Martinson, K. (Year). *Wound Management: Principles and Practices*. 3rd Edition. Healing Arts Press.

- Carter, B. & Roberts, J. (Year). *Infection Control in Wound Care*. Infection Prevention Society.

This chapter provides a comprehensive overview of the foundational principles of wound management, focusing on effective techniques for cleansing, debridement, maintaining a moist environment, and managing infection and inflammation. By adopting a holistic, client-centered, and evidence-based approach, healthcare providers can ensure high-quality care and optimal healing outcomes for their patients.

Chapter 6: Dressings and Wound Care Products

Learning Objectives

By the end of this chapter, you will be able to:

1. Identify and describe various types of dressings and their specific applications in wound care.

2. Understand recent advances in wound care materials, including hydrocolloids, foam dressings, and alginates.

3. Make informed decisions about product selection based on wound type and healing stage.

4. Implement a holistic, client-centered, and evidence-based approach to selecting and applying wound care products.

Overview of Dressing Types and Their Applications

This section provides a comprehensive overview of different types of dressings and their primary uses in wound care:

- **Film Dressings:** Thin, transparent sheets that provide a moisture barrier while allowing the wound to breathe.

- **Hydrogel Dressings:** Provide hydration to dry wounds, promote granulation and autolytic debridement.

- **Hydrocolloid Dressings:** Gel-forming agents that interact with wound exudate to create a moist environment and promote healing.

- **Foam Dressings:** Highly absorbent, providing thermal insulation and moisture control, suitable for wounds with high exudate.

- **Alginate Dressings:** Made from seaweed, highly absorbent, ideal for wounds with significant drainage and for packing wound cavities.

Advances in Wound Care Materials

Technological advancements have significantly improved the functionality and effectiveness of wound care products:

- **Hydrocolloids:** These dressings form a gel as they absorb wound exudate, maintaining a moist environment that accelerates epithelialization.

- **Foam Dressings:** Recent developments have improved their absorptive capacity and reduced their adhesive properties to protect the skin surrounding wounds.

- **Alginates:** New formulations have enhanced their hemostatic properties (ability to stop bleeding), making them more suitable for traumatic and post-surgical wounds.

Product Selection Based on Wound Type and Stage

Choosing the right wound care product is crucial and should be based on the specific characteristics of the wound:

Recommended Treatments for Common Wound Types

1. Pressure Ulcers

- **Dressing Selection:** Foam dressings or hydrocolloids are typically used for pressure ulcers to maintain a moist healing environment and provide cushioning.

- **Rationale:** These dressings help in managing exudate and protect the wound from further injury caused by pressure.

- **Client Education:** Patients should be advised on the importance of regular position changes to relieve pressure and the necessity of maintaining good nutrition to support wound healing.

2. Diabetic Foot Ulcers

- **Dressing Selection:** Alginate dressings or hydrogels can be effective, depending on the exudate level.

- **Rationale:** Alginates are suitable for wounds with significant exudate, while hydrogels keep the wound moist to promote healing in drier ulcers.

- **Client Education:** Education should focus on proper foot care, regular inspection of the feet for wounds or injuries, and controlling blood glucose levels to enhance healing.

3. Venous Ulcers

- **Dressing Selection:** Compression dressings or multilayer compression wraps.

- **Rationale:** Compression therapy is crucial for venous ulcers as it helps reduce edema and improve venous return.

- **Client Education:** Patients should be informed about the importance of leg elevation and wearing compression garments as prescribed. Regular exercise, as tolerated, can also improve circulation.

4. Surgical Wounds

- **Dressing Selection:** Transparent film dressings or hydrocolloid dressings.
- **Rationale:** These dressings allow for monitoring of the surgical site without the need to remove the dressing, which can protect the wound from infection and facilitate faster healing.
- **Client Education:** Educate on signs of infection, the importance of keeping the wound dry and clean, and when to notify healthcare providers of any concerns.

5. Traumatic Wounds

- **Dressing Selection:** Hydrogel or foam dressings, depending on the wound's exudate level.
- **Rationale:** Hydrogel dressings are ideal for wounds with necrotic tissue, promoting autolytic debridement and moist healing. Foam dressings are used when moderate to high exudate is present.
- **Client Education:** Instruction should include how to clean the wound properly, change dressings, and recognize signs of infection.

6. Burns

- **Dressing Selection:** Hydrogel dressings are commonly used for minor burns; more severe burns might require specialized burn dressings like silver sulfadiazine cream or biosynthetic dressings.

- **Rationale:** Hydrogel dressings cool the wound, relieve pain, and donate moisture. Silver dressings help prevent infection in more severe cases.

- **Client Education:** Burns patients should be educated on the need to maintain hydration of the dressing and skin, pain management techniques, and signs of infection. For severe burns, patient education may also include care for skin grafts and prevention of scarring.

Implementing Client-Centered Care

In all cases, treatments should be tailored to each patient's specific needs, taking into account their overall health, lifestyle, and preferences. This approach ensures that wound care management is not only effective in terms of healing but also aligns with the patient's daily life and enhances their overall well-being.

- **Assessing the Wound:** Evaluate the level of exudate, presence of infection, and wound depth.

- **Stage of Healing:** Select products that support the specific phase of healing—whether maintaining moisture for dry wounds, absorbing excess fluid, or protecting new tissue.

- **Patient Comfort and Lifestyle:** Consider ease of application and removal, as well as the patient's activity level and comfort.

Applying a Holistic, Client-Centered, and Evidence-Based Care Model

Selecting the appropriate dressing involves more than just assessing the wound—it requires a holistic approach that considers the entire patient's health, preferences, and lifestyle. This approach ensures that care is personalized and that the chosen products align with evidence-based practices to optimize healing.

Summary of Lessons Learned

- Effective wound management requires a thorough understanding of the various types of dressings and their specific uses.

- Advances in materials technology have broadened the options available, making it possible to tailor treatments to the unique needs of each wound.

- A holistic, client-centered approach in product selection enhances patient satisfaction and outcomes.

References

- Turner, T.D. & White, J.Q. *Modern Wound Dressings: A Clinical Guide*. Wound Care Alliance.

- Patel, G. & Smith, L. *Advances in Wound Care Materials*. TechMed Publications.

This chapter equips healthcare providers with the knowledge needed to navigate the complex array of wound dressings and care products, ensuring that each patient receives the most appropriate and effective treatment tailored to their specific wound care needs.

Chapter 7: Advanced Wound Care Techniques

Learning Objectives

By the end of this chapter, you will be able to:

1. Understand the principles and applications of Negative Pressure Wound Therapy (NPWT).

2. Explain the benefits and uses of Hyperbaric Oxygen Therapy in wound healing.

3. Describe the role of bioengineered skin and tissue products in advanced wound care.

4. Apply a holistic, client-centered, and evidence-based approach to selecting and implementing advanced wound care techniques.

Negative Pressure Wound Therapy (NPWT)

Negative Pressure Wound Therapy involves the use of a vacuum dressing to promote healing in acute or chronic wounds and enhance healing of second and third-degree burns. The section covers:

- **Mechanism of Action:** How NPWT helps by drawing out fluid from the wound and increasing blood flow to the area.

- **Clinical Applications:** Specific scenarios where NPWT has proven beneficial, such as diabetic ulcers and complex soft tissue wounds.

- **Practical Considerations:** Guidelines for setup, monitoring, and managing NPWT, including potential complications.

Negative Pressure Wound Therapy (NPWT) is an advanced wound care therapy that uses a vacuum dressing to promote healing in various types of wounds, including acute, chronic, and second and third-degree burns. Here is an expansion of the considerations, interventions, client education, contraindications, and application tips for NPWT:

Mechanism of Action

- **How NPWT Works:** NPWT aids healing by applying controlled negative pressure (suction) to the wound surface. This vacuum effect helps to reduce edema, draw out excess fluid, decrease bacterial load, and increase blood flow to the area. These factors combined accelerate the formation of granulation tissue.

Clinical Applications

- **Where NPWT is Beneficial:**
    - **Diabetic Ulcers:** Promotes faster healing by improving local circulation and reducing edema.
    - **Complex Soft Tissue Wounds:** Useful in managing wounds that are difficult to heal due to their location or depth.
    - **Surgical Wounds:** Especially those with a high risk of infection or healing complications.
    - **Pressure Ulcers:** Helps in managing large, deep ulcers that do not respond well to other treatments.

Nursing Considerations

- **Patient Assessment:** Evaluate the wound thoroughly before initiating NPWT. Ensure that the therapy is suitable based on wound type and patient condition.

- **Monitoring:** Regular monitoring is crucial to assess the progress of wound healing and identify any signs of infection or other complications.

Nursing Interventions

- **Device Setup and Management:** Proper setup of the NPWT system is essential. This includes securing the dressing, ensuring that the sealing is airtight, and setting the appropriate pressure based on the wound type and location.

- **Regular Inspections:** Check the integrity of the dressing and the device settings regularly to ensure effective therapy.

Client Education

- **Understanding NPWT:** Explain to patients how NPWT works and its benefits. Ensure they understand the importance of device maintenance and alerts.

- **Activity Recommendations:** Advise on activity restrictions or modifications to prevent accidental dislodging of the device.

Contraindications

- **When to Avoid NPWT:**
    - Malignancy in the wound.
    - Untreated osteomyelitis.
    - Exposed blood vessels or nerves.

o Presence of an unexplored fistula.

Application Tips

- **Sealing Techniques:** Use appropriate sealing materials to prevent air leaks, which can compromise the therapy's effectiveness.

- **Pain Management:** Be proactive in managing pain related to NPWT, as the negative pressure can cause discomfort.

Practical Considerations

- **Setup:** Follow manufacturer guidelines for setting up the NPWT system. Training on the use of the device is essential for both healthcare providers and patients (or caregivers) involved in daily care.

- **Monitoring for Complications:** Watch for potential complications such as bleeding, infection, or skin irritation around the dressing. Immediate action may be required to address these issues.

- **Documentation:** Keep detailed records of treatment parameters, changes in wound status, and any patient complaints or observations.

Complications Management

- **Managing Pain:** Adjust the suction level if pain is reported, and ensure analgesics are used effectively.

- **Infection Control:** Maintain strict aseptic techniques during dressing changes to prevent infection.

- **Handling Exudate:** Monitor the amount of exudate being collected. Excessive exudate may require more frequent canister changes and possibly adjustments in therapy settings.

By thoroughly understanding and applying these elements of NPWT, nurses can significantly enhance wound healing outcomes, improve patient comfort, and minimize potential complications associated with this therapy.

Hyperbaric Oxygen Therapy (HBOT)

Hyperbaric Oxygen Therapy involves breathing pure oxygen in a pressurized room or tube, which is a well-established treatment for decompression sickness, serious infections, bubbles of air in blood vessels, and wounds that won't heal as a result of diabetes or radiation injury.

- **Therapeutic Benefits:** HBOT increases the amount of oxygen your blood can carry, which temporarily restores normal levels of blood gases and tissue function to promote healing and fight infection.

- **Indications and Contraindications:** Conditions under which HBOT is recommended or avoided, with a focus on its integration into a comprehensive wound management plan.

Bioengineered Skin and Tissue Products

This technology represents a breakthrough in treating wounds that fail to heal using traditional methods. This section details:

- **Types of Products:** Different types of bioengineered products available, such as cultured skin substitutes and composite skin grafts.

- **Clinical Efficacy:** Discuss how these products provide a permanent or temporary covering to help heal deep wounds and ulcers, reduce the need for skin grafts, and serve as a test-bed for drug interactions.

- **Implementation Guidelines:** Best practices for applying these products, patient selection criteria, and expected outcomes.

Bioengineered skin and tissue products represent a significant advancement in wound care, particularly for treating complex wounds that do not respond to conventional treatment methods. This technology includes a range of products such as cultured skin substitutes, composite skin grafts, and dermal regenerators. Here is an expansion on the types of products, their clinical efficacy, and practical implementation, including nursing considerations, interventions, and client education.

Types of Bioengineered Products

- **Cultured Skin Substitutes:** These are laboratory-grown skin cells that aim to mimic natural skin. They can be derived from the patient's own cells (autologous) or from donor cells (allogeneic).

- **Composite Skin Grafts:** These products are complex structures that include both dermal and epidermal elements. They are designed to provide a more functional and cosmetic match to the native skin.

- **Dermal Regenerators:** These are used in wounds where the dermal layer has been damaged. They provide a scaffold for the body's own cells to regenerate the dermal layer.

Clinical Efficacy

- **Healing Deep Wounds and Ulcers:** Bioengineered products can significantly accelerate the healing process in chronic wounds and ulcers by providing essential growth factors and a supportive structure that facilitates cell migration and proliferation.

- **Reducing the Need for Traditional Skin Grafts:** These products can minimize the necessity for harvesting skin from other areas of the body, a process that can cause additional pain and scarring.

- **Testing Platform for Drug Interactions:** Some bioengineered tissues are used in research to study how drugs interact with human skin, which can be crucial for developing new treatments.

Nursing Considerations

- **Assessment:** Careful assessment of the wound and the patient's overall health is crucial to determine suitability for bioengineered tissue products.

- **Patient Selection:** Ideal candidates are those with wounds that have not responded to traditional healing methods, have sufficient blood supply to support the graft, and do not have active infections.

Nursing Interventions

- **Preparation and Application:** Prepare the wound bed properly by debriding any necrotic tissue and ensuring the area is clean and free of infection. The application of bioengineered tissue must follow strict aseptic techniques.

- **Monitoring:** Regularly monitor the wound for signs of infection, rejection, or failure of the graft to integrate. Assess for adequate blood supply and healing progression.

Client Education

- **Understanding the Product:** Educate patients on the type of bioengineered skin or tissue being used, including how it works and what to expect during the healing process.

- **Care at Home:** Instruct patients on how to care for the wound post-application, such as maintaining a clean environment, recognizing signs of infection, and when to contact healthcare providers.

- **Lifestyle Adjustments:** Discuss any necessary adjustments to lifestyle or activities that might impact the healing process, like nutrition, mobility, and avoiding smoking.

Implementation Guidelines

- **Best Practices:** Follow manufacturer guidelines strictly for storage, preparation, and application of the product. Ensure all handling is done under sterile conditions to prevent contamination.

- **Patient Selection Criteria:** Select patients based on wound characteristics, overall health status, and potential for wound healing. Patients with poor nutritional status or uncontrolled diabetes may need additional interventions to improve outcomes.

- **Expected Outcomes:** Set realistic expectations with patients regarding the time frame for healing and potential outcomes. Ensure they understand the follow-up regimen and any signs of complications to monitor.

Practical Application Tips

- **Follow-Up Care:** Schedule regular follow-up appointments to assess the integration of the graft and overall healing of the wound.

- **Documentation:** Maintain thorough documentation of all aspects of patient care related to the use of bioengineered skin and tissue products, including the specific product used, application details, and patient response.

By integrating these advanced products into clinical practice with careful consideration and patient education, nurses can play a pivotal role in enhancing wound healing outcomes and improving the quality of life for patients with difficult-to-heal wounds.

Applying a Holistic, Client-Centered, and Evidence-Based Care Model

In advanced wound care, a holistic approach not only focuses on the wound itself but also considers the patient's overall physiological and psychological state, lifestyle, and care preferences. This comprehensive care strategy ensures that advanced technologies are used effectively and ethically.

Summary of Lessons Learned

- Advanced wound care techniques such as NPWT, HBOT, and bioengineered products play a critical role in managing complex wound scenarios.

- Successful integration of these technologies into patient care plans requires a thorough understanding of their mechanisms, benefits, and practical applications.

- A holistic, evidence-based approach to advanced wound care enhances healing outcomes and patient satisfaction.

References

- Johnson, M.K., & Lee, A.H. *Advanced Technologies in Wound Care Treatments*. Springer.
- Carter, B.G., & Edwards, H.E. *Clinical Guide to Wound Care and Regeneration*. Elsevier.

This chapter provides an in-depth look at cutting-edge wound care technologies, equipping healthcare professionals with the knowledge and skills needed to implement these advanced techniques effectively and enhance patient care outcomes in complex wound management scenarios.

Chapter 8: Pain Management in Wound Care

Learning Objectives

By the end of this chapter, you will be able to:

1. Understand the physiological and psychological aspects of pain in patients with wounds.

2. Implement both pharmacological and non-pharmacological strategies for effective pain management in wound care.

3. Educate patients and their families on managing pain associated with wound care.

4. Integrate a holistic, client-centered, and evidence-based approach to pain management in the treatment plan.

Understanding Pain in Wound Care Patients

Pain is a common and significant concern in patients with wounds, affecting their quality of life and recovery. This section explores:

- **Types of Pain:** Acute vs. chronic pain and how they relate to different wound types.

- **Pain Assessment:** Techniques and tools for assessing pain intensity and impact, including visual analog scales and pain diaries.

- **Impact of Pain:** Discussion on how pain can affect healing processes, patient mobility, and psychological well-being.

Pharmacological Pain Management Strategies

Effective pharmacological interventions are essential for managing pain in wound care patients. This includes:

- **Topical Analgesics:** Use of local anesthetics or topical NSAIDs directly on or around the wound site.

- **Systemic Medications:** Guidelines for prescribing oral analgesics, such as acetaminophen, NSAIDs, and opioids, based on pain severity and patient condition.

- **Adjuvant Medications:** Utilization of antidepressants, anticonvulsants, and corticosteroids for managing chronic pain associated with wound care.

Effective pain management is a cornerstone of comprehensive wound care, ensuring patient comfort and facilitating better healing outcomes. A multimodal approach often includes topical analgesics, systemic medications, and adjuvant therapies. Here's an expanded look at these interventions, including nursing considerations, interventions, and client education.

Topical Analgesics

Description: Topical analgesics include local anesthetics and topical NSAIDs that can be applied directly to or around the wound to relieve pain without the systemic side effects often associated with oral medications.

Nursing Considerations:

- Assess the wound and surrounding skin integrity before application to avoid adverse reactions.

- Monitor for local allergic reactions or skin irritation.

Nursing Interventions:

- Apply as directed, typically during dressing changes to minimize pain associated with wound manipulation.

- Educate patients on the proper application techniques to ensure effective use.

Client Education:

- Inform patients about possible sensations (e.g., cooling, burning) upon application and what signs to watch for in case of an allergic reaction.

- Emphasize the importance of using these medications as directed to avoid skin damage or reduced effectiveness.

Systemic Medications

Description: Systemic medications include oral analgesics like acetaminophen, NSAIDs, and opioids, which are prescribed based on the severity of pain and overall patient condition.

Nursing Considerations:

- Evaluate the patient's pain level using a standardized pain scale and their overall health to choose an appropriate medication.

- Be mindful of potential side effects, especially gastrointestinal issues with NSAIDs and the risk of addiction or sedation with opioids.

Nursing Interventions:

- Administer medications on a regular schedule or as needed based on the pain assessment.

- Monitor patient response to medications and adjust dosages or medications as necessary in collaboration with the healthcare provider.

Client Education:

- Explain the purpose, potential side effects, and correct usage of each prescribed medication.
- Discuss the importance of not exceeding recommended dosages, especially with opioids and NSAIDs.

Adjuvant Medications

Description: Adjuvant medications, such as antidepressants, anticonvulsants, and corticosteroids, are used for managing chronic pain that might not be fully alleviated by standard analgesics.

Nursing Considerations:

- Consider these medications for patients with neuropathic pain or when pain persists despite other analgesic therapies.
- Monitor for side effects specific to each class of medication, such as dizziness, dry mouth, or potential mood changes.

Nursing Interventions:

- Coordinate with physicians to initiate and adjust these therapies as part of a broader pain management plan.
- Regularly reassess pain and adjust treatment plans based on patient feedback and clinical outcomes.

Client Education:

- Educate patients on how these medications work and why they are being used for wound-related pain.

- Highlight the importance of adherence to prescribed therapies and reporting any adverse effects.

General Tips for Managing Wound Pain:

- Encourage non-pharmacological interventions like relaxation techniques, adequate positioning, and distraction.

- Maintain open communication lines with patients to reassess pain management strategies and adapt as necessary.

Effective pharmacological intervention requires careful consideration of the patient's specific needs, potential risks, and benefits of each medication. By integrating these aspects into pain management protocols, nurses can significantly improve patient comfort and enhance the overall healing process.

Non-Pharmacological Pain Management Strategies

Non-pharmacological methods are vital for a holistic pain management approach. Key strategies include:

- **Physical Methods:** Techniques such as cold and heat therapy, ultrasound, and electrical stimulation to reduce pain perception.

- **Psychological Approaches:** Cognitive-behavioral therapy, relaxation techniques, and biofeedback to help patients cope with pain.

- **Lifestyle Modifications:** Encouraging nutritional support, adequate hydration, and sleep, all of which are crucial for pain management and wound healing.

Non-pharmacological pain management strategies are integral components of a holistic approach to managing pain, particularly in wound care, where pain can be a significant barrier to healing. By incorporating physical methods, psychological approaches, and lifestyle modifications, healthcare providers can support more comprehensive pain relief that enhances the overall quality of life for patients. Here's an expansion on these strategies, including nursing considerations, interventions, and client education:

Physical Methods

Nursing Considerations:

- Assess the patient's overall condition and specific wound characteristics to determine the suitability of physical methods like cold and heat therapy, ultrasound, or electrical stimulation.

- Monitor the patient's response to these therapies to avoid adverse effects, such as burns from heat applications or additional pain from improperly used electrical stimulation.

Nursing Interventions:

- Apply cold therapy for acute injuries to reduce swelling and numb the pain. Heat therapy may be more appropriate for chronic pain to improve blood flow and relax muscles.

- Facilitate the use of ultrasound or TENS (Transcutaneous Electrical Nerve Stimulation) units under appropriate guidance to ensure safety and effectiveness.

Client Education:

- Instruct patients on the proper use of heat and cold therapies, including duration and frequency to prevent skin damage.

- Explain how electrical stimulation works and the sensations they might experience during treatment.

Psychological Approaches

Nursing Considerations:

- Evaluate the patient's emotional and psychological state to tailor psychological interventions effectively. Recognize signs of anxiety, depression, or stress that may exacerbate pain perception.

- Collaborate with mental health professionals when implementing therapies like cognitive-behavioral therapy (CBT) or biofeedback.

Nursing Interventions:

- Implement relaxation techniques such as guided imagery, deep breathing exercises, or progressive muscle relaxation during wound care procedures to help reduce pain perception.

- Support the inclusion of CBT by referring to or working alongside psychologists to help patients develop coping strategies for chronic pain.

Client Education:

- Teach relaxation techniques that patients can use at home.

- Educate about the benefits of psychological interventions in managing pain and the importance of an optimistic outlook on the healing process.

Lifestyle Modifications

Nursing Considerations:

- Assess dietary intake, hydration status, and sleep patterns as part of a comprehensive approach to pain management. Poor nutrition, dehydration, and lack of sleep can all exacerbate pain.

- Consider patient-specific factors such as comorbidities, existing dietary restrictions, and lifestyle when recommending modifications.

Nursing Interventions:

- Encourage balanced diets rich in vitamins and minerals that support healing and potentially reduce pain. A dietitian may provide personalized advice.

- Promote regular, moderate physical activity as tolerated to enhance endorphin production, which naturally alleviates pain.

Client Education:

- Provide guidance on nutritional choices that support wound healing and pain reduction, such as foods rich in omega-3 fatty acids, antioxidants, and protein.

- Advise on the importance of hydration and its role in overall health and pain management.

- Discuss sleep hygiene practices to improve sleep quality, which can influence pain levels.

General Tips for Implementation:

- Always use a patient-centered approach, considering the individual's specific needs, preferences, and capabilities when choosing and implementing non-pharmacological strategies.

- Regularly evaluate the effectiveness of implemented strategies and make adjustments as necessary to optimize outcomes.

By integrating these non-pharmacological strategies into pain management protocols, nurses can provide patients with tools that empower them to actively manage their pain, potentially reducing their reliance on medications and enhancing their overall well-being.

Patient Education on Pain Management

Educating patients and their caregivers about pain management is crucial for compliance and effective care. Education focuses on:

- **Understanding Pain:** Helping patients recognize normal versus abnormal pain during the healing process.

- **Self-Management Techniques:** Teaching patients how to use pain management tools and strategies at home.

- **Communication:** Encouraging open dialogue about pain between patients, caregivers, and healthcare providers.

Mindfulness in Pain Management

Nursing Considerations:

- Evaluate the patient's openness to mindfulness practices. Understanding the patient's attitude towards alternative pain management techniques is crucial for successful implementation.

- Monitor the patient's response to mindfulness exercises to tailor practices to their specific needs, ensuring they are both effective and comfortable.

Nursing Interventions:

- Provide a quiet, comfortable space for the practice of mindfulness exercises, where the patient will not be disturbed.
- Guide the patient through mindfulness sessions or collaborate with a therapist trained in mindfulness-based stress reduction.

Client Education:

- Educate patients on the benefits of mindfulness, which include not only reduced perception of pain but also lowered anxiety levels, improved mood, and enhanced overall well-being.
- Encourage regular practice, explaining that like any skill, mindfulness gets easier and more effective with practice.

Sample Mindfulness Exercise for Pain Relief: Mindful Breathing

Objective: This exercise helps patients focus on their breath, which is a central point of focus in mindfulness practice, helping to divert attention away from pain and induce a state of calm.

Instructions:

1. **Find a Comfortable Position:** Sit in a comfortable chair or lie down in a quiet space. Close your eyes if it helps you focus.

2. **Observe Your Breath:** Pay attention to your natural breathing pattern. Notice the air entering through your nostrils, filling your lungs, and leaving your body. Don't try to change your breathing pattern; simply observe it.

3. **Focus on the Sensation of Breathing:** Feel the sensation of each breath as it enters and exits your nose. Notice the rise and fall of your chest or belly as you breathe.

4. **Acknowledge Pain:** If you notice pain sensations, acknowledge them without judgment. Imagine the breath flowing to and from the area of pain. Each time you breathe out, envision the pain leaving your body with the breath.

5. **Gently Redirect:** Whenever your mind wanders to other thoughts, gently bring your attention back to your breath. It's natural for the mind to wander—part of mindfulness is noticing when it does and gently returning to breathing.

6. **Continue for Several Minutes:** Aim to continue this exercise for 5-10 minutes. As you become more comfortable with the practice, you can extend the duration.

Benefits:

- Helps in detaching from pain by focusing on breathing.

- Induces relaxation and reduces stress, which can exacerbate pain sensations.

- Enhances mental clarity by reducing the clutter of negative thoughts associated with chronic pain.

Client Education Tips:

- Encourage daily practice, ideally at the same time each day, to establish a routine.

- Advise patients that it's normal for the mind to wander and that the skill of mindfulness grows with practice.

- Recommend starting with short sessions and gradually increasing their duration as comfort with the practice grows.

Incorporating mindfulness into pain management provides a powerful tool for patients, empowering them to take an active role in managing their pain. It's beneficial not only for physical pain relief but also for enhancing emotional resilience in coping with chronic pain conditions.

Applying a Holistic, Client-Centered, and Evidence-Based Care Model

Adopting a comprehensive approach ensures that all aspects of the patient's health and well-being are considered when managing pain. This approach emphasizes personalized care plans that address both physical and emotional aspects of wound-related pain.

Summary of Lessons Learned

- Effective pain management in wound care requires an understanding of pain types and comprehensive assessment techniques.

- Integrating pharmacological and non-pharmacological strategies is crucial for managing pain effectively.

- Educating patients and their families on pain management techniques enhances patient autonomy and improves care outcomes.

References

- Smith, J., & Brown, C. (Year). *Pain Management in Wound Care*. Healing Press.

- Johnson, M., & Lee, T. (Year). *Holistic Approaches to Pain in Wound Management*. Medical Wisdom Press.

This chapter provides detailed insights into understanding and managing pain in wound care patients, emphasizing the importance of a holistic, patient-centered approach that leverages both pharmacological and non-pharmacological strategies to enhance patient comfort and facilitate healing.

Chapter 9: Nutritional Considerations in Wound Healing

Learning Objectives

By the end of this chapter, you will be able to:

1. Understand the role of nutrition in the wound healing process.

2. Conduct nutritional assessments to identify deficiencies impacting wound healing.

3. Implement nutritional interventions tailored to enhance wound healing.

4. Analyze case studies to apply nutritional knowledge in practical wound care settings.

5. Utilize a holistic, client-centered, and evidence-based approach to integrate nutrition into wound care management.

Nutrition's Role in Wound Healing

Nutrition plays a critical role in wound healing, providing the necessary nutrients that support cellular activities essential for repair processes. This section explores:

- **Macronutrients and Micronutrients:** The importance of proteins, carbohydrates, fats, vitamins (such as A, C, and E), and minerals (like zinc and iron) in collagen synthesis, immune function, and tissue regeneration.

- **Energy Requirements:** Understanding the increased caloric needs of wound healing patients to support the metabolic demands of recovery.

Proper nutrition plays a crucial role in wound healing, as it supports the body's repair mechanisms, boosts immune function, and enhances tissue regeneration. Here's an expanded overview of the importance of macronutrients and micronutrients, as well as energy requirements, with a focus on nursing considerations, interventions, and client education.

Macronutrients and Micronutrients

Nursing Considerations:

- Assess the patient's dietary intake and nutritional status to identify any deficiencies that may impede wound healing.

- Monitor patients with wounds for signs of malnutrition or specific nutrient deficiencies, which can delay healing processes.

Nursing Interventions:

- Collaborate with dietitians to develop a nutrition plan that meets the individual dietary needs of patients, focusing on increasing intake of essential nutrients.

- Administer supplements as prescribed to address specific deficiencies.

Client Education:

- **Proteins:** Essential for collagen synthesis and immune function. Educate patients on sources of high-quality protein like lean meats, eggs, and legumes.

- **Carbohydrates:** Provide the necessary energy to fuel the healing process. Emphasize the importance of complex carbohydrates, such as whole grains, for sustained energy.

- **Fats:** Important for cellular function and as carriers for fat-soluble vitamins. Advise on healthy fats sources like avocados, nuts, and olive oil.

- **Vitamins:**

    - *Vitamin A:* Supports immune function and is crucial for cellular growth. Found in dairy products, carrots, and leafy greens.

    - *Vitamin C:* Essential for collagen synthesis and is an antioxidant. Sources include citrus fruits, peppers, and strawberries.

    - *Vitamin E:* Helps protect cell membranes and supports immune health. Found in nuts, seeds, and vegetable oils.

- **Minerals:**

    - *Zinc:* Plays a role in collagen synthesis, protein synthesis, and cellular proliferation. Sources include meat, shellfish, and legumes.

    - *Iron:* Essential for oxygen transport in the blood, supporting energy levels. Found in red meat, fortified cereals, and spinach.

Energy Requirements

Nursing Considerations:

- Understand that patients with wounds have increased metabolic demands and may require additional calories to support the healing process.

- Monitor weight, muscle mass, and overall energy levels to adjust dietary intake as needed.

Nursing Interventions:

- Calculate the energy needs of wound healing patients, which can be significantly higher than the standard dietary recommendations.

- Ensure that meals are calorie-dense and nutrient-rich to meet the increased energy demands without requiring large volumes of food, which might be difficult for some patients to consume.

Client Education:

- Educate patients on the importance of meeting their increased caloric needs through balanced meals.

- Discuss meal planning and snacking on healthy, high-calorie foods to boost energy intake throughout the day.

- Highlight the significance of regular meal times and not skipping meals to maintain a consistent energy supply for healing.

General Tips for Implementation:

- Regularly reassess the nutritional status and adjust dietary plans as the patient progresses through different stages of wound healing.

- Encourage patients to keep a food diary to monitor their intake and adjust their diet based on observed impacts on their energy levels and wound healing progress.

By integrating these nutritional considerations into wound care management, nurses can significantly influence healing outcomes. Effective nutrition education empowers patients to make informed choices that support their recovery, promoting faster and more effective wound healing.

Nutritional Assessments and Interventions

Effective nutritional management starts with a thorough assessment followed by tailored interventions. Key components include:

- **Nutritional Screening:** Identifying at-risk patients using tools like the Mini Nutritional Assessment.

- **Dietary Analysis:** Evaluating dietary intake to spot potential nutrient gaps.

- **Intervention Strategies:** Developing dietary plans that include nutrient-rich foods and supplementation to meet the specific needs of wound healing patients.

Nutritional assessments and interventions are critical components of comprehensive care, particularly in managing patients with wounds. Proper nutrition significantly influences the healing process, impacting everything from immune function to tissue repair. Here's an expanded overview of the process, including interdisciplinary considerations, nutritional screening, dietary analysis, and intervention strategies.

Nutritional Screening

Interdisciplinary Considerations:

- Collaborate with dietitians, physicians, and nursing staff to identify patients at risk of malnutrition or specific nutrient deficiencies.

- Use standardized tools such as the Mini Nutritional Assessment (MNA) to systematically evaluate nutritional status. This tool is especially useful in geriatric populations where malnutrition risks are higher.

Nursing Interventions:

- Regularly screen patients upon admission and periodically throughout their care, especially if there is a change in their condition or treatment plan that might affect nutritional status.

- Document and communicate any findings that suggest a risk of malnutrition to the broader healthcare team.

Client Education:

- Educate patients and caregivers about the importance of nutrition in wound healing and overall health.

- Discuss the signs of malnutrition (e.g., weight loss, fatigue, decreased muscle strength) to ensure they understand when to seek further evaluation or help.

Dietary Analysis

Interdisciplinary Considerations:

- Work closely with dietitians to analyze dietary intakes and identify gaps. Dietitians can provide specialized knowledge in assessing nutrient intake accurately.

- Consider the input from occupational therapists if physical limitations affect the patient's ability to eat (e.g., difficulty swallowing or limited hand dexterity).

Nursing Interventions:

- Collect detailed dietary histories to understand the patient's usual intake patterns and preferences.
- Assess the patient's ability to access and prepare food, as socioeconomic factors can impact nutritional status.

Client Education:

- Instruct patients on how to keep a food diary to accurately track their dietary intake, which can be analyzed by healthcare providers to identify specific needs.
- Provide practical tips on preparing nutrient-rich meals, possibly in collaboration with occupational therapists if modifications to kitchen tools or techniques are needed.

Intervention Strategies

Interdisciplinary Considerations:

- Integrate advice from dietitians, wound care specialists, and pharmacists to coordinate nutritional supplements with other medical treatments.
- Ensure that any dietary recommendations consider existing medical conditions (e.g., diabetes, renal disease) and the overall treatment objectives for each patient.

Nursing Interventions:

- Implement dietary changes and supplementation based on assessment results. For example, increasing protein intake in patients with pressure ulcers or enhancing vitamin C intake in those with surgical wounds.

- Monitor the effectiveness of the dietary interventions on wound healing and adjust as necessary.

Client Education:

- Explain how specific nutrients affect wound healing. For example, protein is essential for tissue repair, while vitamin C helps in collagen formation.

- Discuss the role of hydration in healing and overall health, emphasizing the need to balance fluid intake, especially in patients with kidney or heart conditions.

General Implementation Tips:

- Regular follow-ups to reassess the patient's nutritional status and adapt interventions as the patient's condition evolves.

- Foster a collaborative atmosphere where patients feel supported in asking questions and expressing concerns about their dietary needs or preferences.

Effective nutritional management in wound care requires a well-coordinated approach among various healthcare professionals. By conducting thorough assessments and tailoring interventions to meet individual needs, the interdisciplinary team can significantly enhance patient outcomes and accelerate the healing process.

Case Studies on Nutrition Management

This section presents detailed case studies illustrating successful nutritional management strategies in wound care:

- **Case Study 1:** Management of a diabetic patient with a foot ulcer, focusing on glycemic control and protein supplementation.

- **Case Study 2:** Nutritional intervention for a pressure ulcer patient in a long-term care facility, highlighting the role of hydration and micronutrient supplementation.

- **Case Study 3:** Addressing malnutrition in a post-surgical wound patient through enteral feeding.

Case Study 1: Management of a Diabetic Patient with a Foot Ulcer

Nursing Considerations:

- Monitor the patient's blood glucose levels regularly to ensure tight glycemic control, which is crucial in healing diabetic ulcers.

- Assess dietary intake to ensure sufficient protein which is essential for wound healing.

Nursing Interventions:

- Coordinate with a dietitian to create a meal plan that balances the patient's diabetic needs with increased protein requirements.

- Educate the patient on the importance of foot care and regular inspection to prevent further injury.

Client Education:

- Teach the patient how to monitor their blood sugar levels and discuss the impact of glycemic control on wound healing.

- Provide information on protein-rich foods suitable for diabetics and encourage consistent dietary habits.

Reflective Questions:

- How might fluctuating blood glucose levels affect the healing of a diabetic foot ulcer?

- What steps can the patient take to integrate regular foot inspections into their daily routine?

Case Study 2: Nutritional Intervention for a Pressure Ulcer Patient in a Long-Term Care Facility

Nursing Considerations:

- Regularly assess the patient's hydration status as dehydration can slow wound healing and is a common issue in long-term care settings.

- Monitor micronutrient levels, particularly focusing on vitamins and minerals crucial for skin integrity and healing.

Nursing Interventions:

- Implement a hydration protocol, ensuring the patient receives adequate fluids throughout the day.

- Work with a dietitian to supplement the patient's diet with key micronutrients like vitamin C, zinc, and iron.

Client Education:

- Educate the patient and care staff on the signs of dehydration and the importance of regular fluid intake.
- Discuss the role of specific micronutrients in wound healing and how dietary choices can impact recovery.

Reflective Questions:

- What challenges might a caregiver face in maintaining adequate hydration for a patient, and how can these be overcome?
- How does micronutrient supplementation contribute to the management of pressure ulcers?

Case Study 3: Addressing Malnutrition in a Post-Surgical Wound Patient Through Enteral Feeding

Nursing Considerations:

- Evaluate the patient's nutritional status to identify specific deficiencies and caloric needs.
- Monitor the patient's tolerance to enteral feeding, watching for potential complications like aspiration or gastrointestinal discomfort.

Nursing Interventions:

- Initiate enteral feeding based on a comprehensive assessment by a nutritionist, tailored to meet the patient's energy and nutrient requirements.
- Regularly reassess the patient's progress in terms of wound healing and adjust the feeding regimen as needed.

Client Education:

- Explain the purpose and process of enteral feeding, including how it will help with wound healing.

- Teach the patient and caregivers about managing the feeding equipment and recognizing signs of potential problems.

Reflective Questions:

- Why is enteral feeding chosen over other nutritional support methods in some post-surgical patients?

- What factors should be considered when tailoring an enteral nutrition plan for a patient with a post-surgical wound?

These case studies illustrate the importance of integrating tailored nutritional management and consistent medical care in treating complex wound conditions. By reflecting on these questions, healthcare providers can better understand the intricate relationship between nutrition and wound healing and improve their care strategies accordingly.

Applying a Holistic, Client-Centered, and Evidence-Based Care Model

Nutritional care in wound healing should consider the entire individual, including their medical history, lifestyle, and personal preferences, ensuring that interventions are patient-centered and grounded in the best available evidence.

Summary of Lessons Learned

- Nutrition is a foundational aspect of effective wound management, crucial for optimal healing.

- Tailored nutritional assessments and interventions are essential to address the unique needs of each patient.

- Real-world case studies demonstrate the practical application and impact of nutritional strategies in wound care.

References

- Thompson, C., & Carter, N. ***Nutritional Guidelines for Wound Healing***. Academic Health Publications.

- Moore, Z., & Jenkins, M. ***Clinical Nutrition for Wound Care Recovery***. Wiley-Blackwell.

This chapter underscores the importance of nutrition in wound healing, providing healthcare professionals with the knowledge and tools needed to assess and address the nutritional needs of patients with wounds effectively. Through a comprehensive understanding and strategic application of nutritional care, clinicians can significantly enhance the healing outcomes and overall health of their patients.

Chapter 10: Ethical and Legal Considerations in Wound Care

Learning Objectives

By the end of this chapter, you will be able to:

1. Identify and analyze ethical dilemmas commonly encountered in wound care nursing.

2. Understand the legal aspects related to wound care treatment and documentation.

3. Apply knowledge of case law and precedents to wound care practices.

4. Integrate a holistic, client-centered, and evidence-based approach to navigate ethical and legal challenges in wound care.

Ethical Dilemmas in Wound Care Nursing

Ethical dilemmas in wound care often arise from conflicting values and duties such as balancing patient autonomy with beneficence. This section discusses:

- **Consent and Autonomy:** Challenges in obtaining informed consent for wound care procedures.

- **Resource Allocation:** Ethical considerations in allocating limited resources, such as advanced dressings and technologies.

- **End-of-Life Care:** Managing wounds in palliative care settings, focusing on comfort versus aggressive treatment.

Legal Aspects of Wound Care Treatment and Documentation

Legal requirements in wound care are critical for compliance and protecting both the patient and healthcare provider. Topics covered include:

- **Documentation Standards:** Detailed recording of wound assessments, treatment plans, and patient interactions to comply with legal standards.
- **Confidentiality and Privacy:** Upholding patient confidentiality in the handling and sharing of medical records.
- **Liability and Negligence:** Understanding legal implications in cases of alleged malpractice or negligence in wound care.

Case Law and Precedent in Wound Care

Illustrative case studies and precedents that have shaped legal practices in wound care include:

- **Case Study 1:** A lawsuit resulting from a failure to prevent pressure ulcers in a nursing home, highlighting the importance of standard care protocols.
- **Case Study 2:** A case involving inadequate documentation of wound progression and treatment, emphasizing the legal ramifications of poor record-keeping.

Applying a Holistic, Client-Centered, and Evidence-Based Care Model

Addressing ethical and legal considerations in wound care requires a comprehensive approach that respects patient rights and adheres to professional standards. This involves:

- **Patient-Centered Care:** Ensuring that care decisions are made with respect to the patient's values, needs, and preferences.

- **Evidence-Based Practice:** Basing care decisions on the latest research and best practices to ensure high standards of care and legal compliance.

Summary of Lessons Learned

- Navigating ethical dilemmas and legal issues is crucial for effective and responsible wound care management.

- Thorough documentation and adherence to legal standards are vital for clinical practice and legal protection.

- Ethical and legal considerations must be integrated into daily practice to uphold quality care and patient safety.

References

- Black, J., & White, S. *Ethics and Law in Wound Care*. Springer.

- Green, M. L., & Johnson, T. R. *Legal Risks in Wound Care*. LegalMed Publications.

This chapter equips wound care professionals with the knowledge to handle ethical challenges and legal responsibilities effectively, ensuring that care practices not only meet clinical requirements but also adhere to ethical standards and legal obligations. This comprehensive approach helps foster a safe, respectful, and legally compliant healthcare environment.

Chapter 11: Interprofessional Wound Care Team

Learning Objectives

By the end of this chapter, you will be able to:

1. Describe the roles and responsibilities of each member of the interprofessional wound care team.

2. Understand the importance of interprofessional collaboration in delivering comprehensive wound care.

3. Analyze case studies that illustrate successful interprofessional team management in wound care settings.

4. Apply a holistic, client-centered, and evidence-based approach to enhance teamwork and patient outcomes in wound care.

Roles and Responsibilities of the Wound Care Team

The effectiveness of wound care often hinges on the coordinated efforts of an interprofessional team. This section outlines:

- **Nurses:** Specialize in day-to-day wound management and patient education.

- **Physicians:** Provide medical oversight, perform surgical interventions, and manage complex cases.

- **Physical Therapists:** Focus on mobility, reducing pressure on wound sites, and enhancing circulation.

- **Dietitians:** Offer nutritional support to promote wound healing.

- **Social Workers:** Assist with the psychosocial aspects of long-term wound management and patient advocacy.

Importance of Interprofessional Collaboration

Collaboration across different specialties is crucial for effective wound care management. Key points include:

- **Holistic Care:** A comprehensive approach ensures all aspects of patient health are addressed, enhancing healing outcomes.

- **Efficiency and Innovation:** Collaborative teams can streamline care processes and innovate treatments through shared expertise.

- **Patient-Centered Outcomes:** Integrating diverse professional insights helps tailor treatments to individual patient needs and preferences.

Case Studies of Successful Team Management

This section presents real-world examples of how effective interprofessional collaboration leads to improved wound care outcomes:

- **Case Study 1:** A diabetic patient with a non-healing foot ulcer treated successfully through coordinated efforts between healthcare providers, including innovative use of new dressing materials and revised nutritional plans.

- **Case Study 2:** Management of a pressure ulcer in an elderly patient that involved nurses, a dietitian, and a physical therapist to optimize care, prevent reoccurrences, and educate the family on supportive care practices at home.

Case Study 1: Successful Treatment of a Diabetic Foot Ulcer

Nursing Considerations:

- **Assessment:** Continuous assessment of the foot ulcer to evaluate healing progress and identify any signs of infection or deterioration. Consider factors like blood glucose levels and nutritional status as integral to the healing process.

- **Interdisciplinary Collaboration:** Coordinate care with various healthcare providers including podiatrists, dietitians, and wound care specialists to apply a comprehensive treatment approach.

Nursing Interventions:

- **Innovative Dressing Use:** Implement new and advanced dressing materials that promote moist wound healing and possibly contain antimicrobial properties. Monitor the wound's response to these dressings and adjust the treatment plan based on observations.

- **Nutritional Revision:** Work with a dietitian to enhance the patient's dietary regimen, focusing on optimizing glycemic control and enriching the diet with nutrients essential for wound healing, such as proteins, vitamins A and C, and zinc.

Client Education:

- Educate the patient on the importance of maintaining consistent blood glucose levels to facilitate wound healing.

- Instruct on proper foot care techniques and the significance of regular monitoring and reporting of any changes in the wound's condition.

Reflective Questions:

- How do changes in dressing materials contribute to wound healing in diabetic patients?

- What role does dietary management play in the healing process of diabetic foot ulcers?

Case Study 2: Comprehensive Management of a Pressure Ulcer in an Elderly Patient

Nursing Considerations:

- **Holistic Care Approach:** Ensure a holistic approach by involving interdisciplinary team members to address all aspects of patient care, including nutritional status, physical mobility, and skin integrity.

- **Risk Assessment:** Regularly assess the patient for risk factors associated with pressure ulcer development, such as mobility limitations and nutritional deficiencies.

Nursing Interventions:

- **Collaborative Care Planning:** Coordinate with a dietitian to optimize nutritional intake that supports skin integrity and healing. Engage a physical therapist to assist with mobility and reducing pressure on vulnerable areas.

- **Family Education:** Train family members in care techniques that prevent pressure ulcer reoccurrences, such as proper positioning, skin inspection, and the use of supportive devices.

Client Education:

- Provide detailed instructions on the daily care routines that help in pressure ulcer prevention and management.

- Educate about the signs of potential complications and when to seek professional help.

Reflective Questions:

- What are the key factors to consider in preventing the recurrence of pressure ulcers in elderly patients?

- How can family involvement be enhanced in the care of a patient with a pressure ulcer?

These case studies emphasize the necessity of a coordinated approach among healthcare professionals to manage complex patient cases effectively. Reflective questions engage the reader in critical thinking about the holistic care processes, the integration of new technologies, and the importance of patient and family education in managing chronic conditions.

Applying a Holistic, Client-Centered, and Evidence-Based Care Model

Emphasizing a team-based approach that considers the whole person — not just the wound — ensures that all factors affecting healing are considered. This approach enhances patient satisfaction and treatment efficacy.

Summary of Lessons Learned

- Effective wound care requires the coordinated efforts of a diverse interprofessional team.

- Collaboration enhances care quality by pooling diverse expertise, leading to innovative and personalized patient care.

- Case studies demonstrate the practical benefits of interprofessional teamwork in real-world settings.

References

- Johnson, M.K., & Lee, A.H. (Year). *Team Approaches in Wound Management*. Springer.

- Carter, B.G., & Edwards, H.E. (Year). *Interprofessional Collaboration in Wound Care*. Elsevier.

This chapter details the critical roles within an interprofessional wound care team and underscores the importance of collaboration in achieving superior patient outcomes. By understanding and implementing effective team dynamics, healthcare professionals can provide more comprehensive and effective wound care.

Chapter 12: Patient Education and Home Care

Learning Objectives

By the end of this chapter, you will be able to:

1. Effectively educate patients and their caregivers on wound care management.

2. Develop comprehensive home care plans that address the specific needs of each patient.

3. Utilize community resources to support patients' wound care outside of clinical settings.

4. Integrate a holistic, client-centered, and evidence-based approach to enhance patient education and home care.

Educating Patients and Caregivers

Effective patient and caregiver education is crucial for the successful management of wounds at home. This section discusses:

- **Understanding Wound Care Basics:** Teaching the fundamentals of wound healing, including how to recognize signs of infection or complications.

- **Instruction on Dressing Changes:** Detailed demonstrations and guidance on how to change dressings, clean wounds, and recognize when medical consultation is needed.

- **Empowering Self-Management:** Providing tools and strategies to enable patients and caregivers to feel confident in managing wound care independently.

Developing Effective Home Care Plans

Home care plans must be tailored to fit the individual needs of patients, ensuring they are practical and sustainable. Key components include:

- **Assessment of Home Environment:** Evaluating the patient's living conditions to adapt the care plan accordingly.

- **Customized Care Guidelines:** Creating personalized care instructions that align with the patient's lifestyle and capabilities.

- **Regular Follow-Up:** Establishing a schedule for regular check-ins either virtually or in person to adjust the care plan as the wound heals.

Utilizing Community Resources for Wound Care

Leveraging community resources can greatly enhance the support available to patients managing wounds at home. This involves:

- **Local Wound Care Clinics:** Guiding patients to accessible local services for periodic professional wound assessments.

- **Support Groups:** Connecting patients with support groups for emotional and practical support from others who are facing similar challenges.

- **Educational Workshops:** Encouraging participation in workshops that teach wound care skills and provide up-to-date information on best practices.

Applying a Holistic, Client-Centered, and Evidence-Based Care Model

Incorporating a comprehensive approach that considers the patient's overall well-being and environment is essential for successful home wound care. This strategy ensures that all aspects of the patient's health and lifestyle are considered in the care plan.

Summary of Lessons Learned

- Effective patient and caregiver education is fundamental to successful wound management at home.

- Personalized home care plans and regular follow-ups are essential to adapt to the changing needs of the wound and patient.

- Community resources play a significant role in supporting ongoing wound care management outside the clinical setting.

References

- Thompson, J., & Davis, M. *Home Wound Care Strategies*. Wiley-Blackwell.

- Allen, L., & Martin, F. *Community Resources for Wound Management*. Community Health Publications.

This chapter outlines the importance of patient education and the development of tailored home care plans, emphasizing the role of community resources in supporting wound care. By educating patients and caregivers effectively and providing them with the necessary tools and support, healthcare professionals can ensure better outcomes and greater patient autonomy in wound management.

Appendices

Appendix A: Quick Reference Charts for Wound Types and Care Options

1. Wound Types and Characteristics

- **Pressure Ulcers:** Location typically over bony prominences, caused by sustained pressure.

- **Diabetic Foot Ulcers:** Commonly located on the foot, result from neuropathy and poor circulation.

- **Venous Ulcers:** Typically found on the lower legs, due to venous insufficiency.

- **Arterial Ulcers:** Located on feet and legs, caused by poor arterial blood flow.

- **Surgical Wounds:** Result from surgical incisions, risk of infection based on procedure type.

- **Traumatic Wounds:** Result from physical injury; can vary widely in type and severity.

- **Burns:** Classified by depth (first, second, third degree), cause (thermal, chemical, electrical).

2. Recommended Care Options

- **Pressure Ulcers:** Pressure relief devices, regular repositioning, moisture management.

- **Diabetic Foot Ulcers:** Off-loading, infection control, blood glucose management.

- **Venous Ulcers:** Compression therapy, elevation of limbs, wound cleansing.

- **Arterial Ulcers:** Revascularization, pain management, protection from trauma.

- **Surgical Wounds:** Sterile dressing changes, monitoring for signs of infection, adequate nutrition.

- **Traumatic Wounds:** Debridement, tetanus prophylaxis, broad-spectrum antimicrobials if indicated.

- **Burns:** Cooling, sterile dressings, pain management, fluid resuscitation for severe cases.

Appendix B: Glossary of Terms

- **Autolytic Debridement:** The use of the body's own mechanisms to remove dead tissue from the wound.

- **Bioburden:** The presence of bacteria on the surface of the wound that does not necessarily cause infection but can affect healing.

- **Collagen:** A protein that is a major component in skin tissue repair.

- **Exudate:** Fluid, such as pus or clear fluid, that leaks out of blood vessels into nearby tissues and is produced by the body in response to infection or inflammation.

- **Granulation Tissue:** New vascular tissue in granular form on an ulcer or the healing surface of a wound.

- **Macrophage:** A type of white blood cell that engulfs and digests cellular debris and pathogens.

- **Necrotic:** Referring to dead tissue that is present in a wound.

- **Revascularization:** The restoration of perfusion to a body part or organ that has suffered ischemia.

- **Shear:** A force that causes layers of tissue to slide over one another, potentially leading to tissue damage and ulcer formation.

About the Author

Chad Peterson, RPN, CFCN

Chad Peterson is a seasoned Registered Practical Nurse and a certified Advanced FootCare Nurse based in Ontario, Canada. With years of dedicated service in the healthcare industry, Chad has specialized in the intricate fields of foot care and wound management. His profound commitment to enhancing patient care through education and practical skills is evident in his work.

Chad is the esteemed author of "Mastering the Art of Footcare Nursing," a comprehensive guide that has served as a pivotal resource for healthcare professionals seeking to deepen their knowledge and expertise in foot care. Building on this foundation, his latest work, "Advanced Wound Care Nursing: Techniques and Management," further cements his status as an expert in both foot care and advanced wound management.

Throughout his career, Chad has pursued numerous advanced courses in wound care, continually updating his skills and staying abreast of the latest advancements in treatment methodologies. His practical experience, combined with an ongoing pursuit of knowledge, allows him to provide exceptional care to his patients and valuable insights to his readers.

Other Publications:

- "Mastering the Art of Footcare Nursing"

Contact Information:

- **LinkedIn:** Chad Peterson, RPN, CFCN

Chad remains deeply committed to the education and advancement of nursing professionals, sharing his expertise through writing, workshops, and seminars. His work not only enlightens fellow healthcare workers but also significantly improves the quality of life for patients under their care.

The Healing Touch: A Tribute to Wound Care Nurses

by Chad Peterson

In the quiet hum of healing wards there lies, A gentle strength beneath the watchful eyes. Nurses tread where wounds and sorrows dwell, In silent battles, stories they will tell.

With hands both tender and wrapped in care, They dress each wound with skill and flare. A touch so light, a whisper soft, Calming fears that soar aloft.

In layers wrapped of gauze and grace, Each bandage placed with measured pace. The art of healing, their silent creed, For every wound, they plant a seed.

Amid the sterile scent and steely rooms, Their presence whispers through the glooms. With every dressing, hope is spun, Underneath the white-clad sun.

They see not just the wound, but the person beneath, Fighting battles with every breath and seethe. Guiding with knowledge, a path they chart, For wound care is science as much as heart.

A nurse stands by with vigil kept, Through restless days and nights unslept. For in each healing curve and scar, Lies a story of resilience, near and far.

Oh, heroes masked in scrubs of blue, To your calling steadfast, ever true. In wound care's tender, meticulous dance, You give the gift of a second chance.

www.ingramcontent.com/pod-product-compliance
Lightning Source LLC
Chambersburg PA
CBHW071200240526
45470CB00017B/664